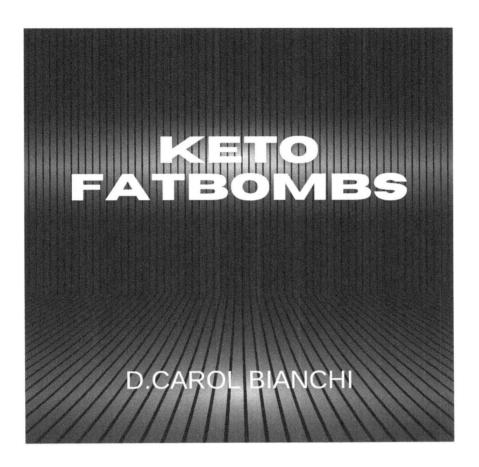

KETO FATBOMBS

D.CAROL BIANCHI

PAGEMAN

1

2

50+ Original Recipes for Fast Weight Loss with Taste

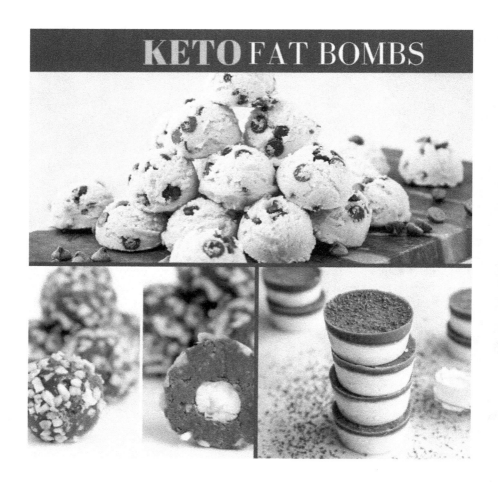

Summary

6

By D. Carol Bianchi

INTRODUCTION

This idea was born from an email from a customer (thank you, Nidza), which went something like this...

'Well I normally fix meals to last me at most four serving or days. I'd plan to have a fat bomb every day.

That's 365 days divided by a recipe that makes at least a weeks' worth, so <u>52 recipes</u>?

<u>That's ideal.</u> Are there 52 fat bomb recipes anywhere?

Perfection in my mind would be a <u>seasonally adjusted book</u> where you would split the recipes into <u>four seasons.</u>

To allow for not always <u>sweet</u> but <u>savory recipes</u> utilizing available produce and lots of fat. How's that *for a crazy idea?'*

And with this 'crazy idea' in mind, I went about to create a range of fat bombs across the seasons. There is a good mixture of sweet and savory, along with some very special holiday themed fat bombs.

This book was perhaps my most challenging and creative yet. So I hope you enjoy these fat bombs and they help you to stay keto by adding a bit of variety and delight to your diet.

As with most things.. everything in moderation. Yes, they are ketogenic, however I would not recommend getting all your daily calories from them. I suggest using them as a treat, perhaps one a day as Nidza has suggested.

D. Carol Bianchi

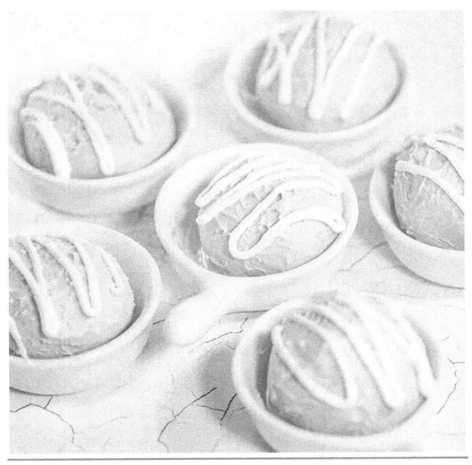

EXAMPLE

When previewing a recipe book on Amazon, I like to be able to view the recipes, rather than the whole "preview" being the introduction or guide. So you can see what you are getting, below is one of the delicious recipes to help decide if you'd like to download the book.

COCONUT LIME FAT BOMBS

Preparation time: 5 minutes
Cooking time: 0 minutes
Makes: 24

INGREDIENTS:

- 1 stick unsalted butter
- ¾ cup coconut oil
- 1 ounce unsweetened, shredded coconut
- Zest and juice of 2 small limes
- 4 ounces cream cheese, softened
- ¼ cup unsweetened coconut cream
- ¼ teaspoon vanilla extract
- Sugar-free sweetener of your choice, to taste

DIRECTIONS:

1. Add the butter and coconut oil to a saucepan and set over medium heat. Once melted, remove from the heat and stir in the lime zest and juice.

2. Stir in the vanilla and shredded coconut. Then add the softened cream cheese and coconut cream. Mix well until the mixture is as smooth as possible. If you notice that the cream cheese has separated, don't worry about that as it won't affect the result. Add the sweetener to your taste and mix well.

3. Spoon the mixture into candy molds or candy paper liners and place in the freezer for about an hour. Once they are set, remove from the molds and enjoy.

4. Store the candies in an airtight container in the freezer.

NUTRITION FACTS (PER SERVING)

Total Carbohydrates: 1g

Dietary Fiber: .0g

Net Cabs: 1g

Protein: 1g

Total Fat: 14g

Calories: 122

OVERVIEW OF THE KETOGENIC DIET

I assume you know a bit, or maybe a lot about the Ketogenic Diet at this point, but just in case, let's have a quick overview of what the Ketogenic Diet is before diving into the recipes.

Our body's metabolism has evolved much less quickly than modern technology. In the past, we had to hunt for our meals and we would often go without food for days or weeks at a time. So our bodies stored as much of its energy reserves as possible for when it was needed. The body became extremely efficient at taking any excess energy (from food) and storing it for later (as fat). When food became scarce, the body would switch from using food as its primary source of energy to the fat reserves.

However, in modern life, food is far more plentiful, but excess energy is still be stored as fat. Modern life has exacerbated this by producing foods rich in carbohydrates (which are utilized more quickly by the body) and lowering the need for physical activity. As a result, excess energy (more calories consumed than expended) is more abundant and consequently more energy is stored (usually as fat).

The concept of the ketogenic diet is that it takes advantage of your body's natural system that uses fat for fuel. By switching to a low carbohydrate diet, your body adapts and becomes unable to utilize the readily available source of carbohydrate that was once available to it. Instead, it begins to use both existing and new stores of fat as its energy source. This is known as a state of ketosis.

When we are on a diet containing sufficient amounts of carbohydrate, these are broken down into glucose which is used for energy. However, when carbs are restricted, our liver starts to produce ketones (also known as ketone bodies). These are transported from the liver to other tissues where they can be reconverted by enzymes in the body to produce energy.

That is the theory behind the diet, and in practice it breaks down into the below macronutrients:

- Carbs - 20 - 50 grams per day
    - Try 30 grams to begin with and see how you feel and are progressing (see measuring results below).
- Protein – 1.5 – 2.6 grams per pound (0.7 – 1.2 grams per kg) of body weight
    - If your level of physical activity is high, go for the higher end as it will help to retain/ build muscle.
- Fat – remaining calories from (healthy) fats.

The above is an overview, but if you would like to know more about the diet in detail, then I have a complete guide to the diet along with how to make it <u>sustainable in the long term</u> - to the point where you no longer have to <u>count calories</u>.

FINAL NOTES

Adjusting and customizing the recipes

These recipes have been created to:

1. Be easy to make
2. Be delicious
3. Use easy to find ingredients

However, there is not a one size fits all recipe, everyone has different tastes, some have allergies and not everyone will be able to get all of the ingredients. Consider the recipes as a guideline to which you can then customize to your taste or to what you have in the house.

- Love coconut? Try coconut flour instead of almond.
- Do not have any pink rock salt in the house? Just use some normal table salt instead.

SPRING

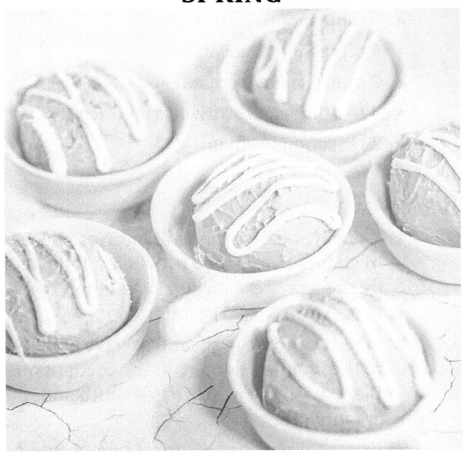

STRAWBERRY FAT BOMBS

Preparation time: 5 minutes
Cooking time: 0 minutes
Serves: 12

INGREDIENTS:

- 4 tablespoons butter
- 4 tablespoons coconut oil
- 2 ounces heavy cream
- 3 regular sized strawberries, diced
- 2 teaspoons Truvia

DIRECTIONS:

1. Wash and dice the strawberries. Place in an blender or food processor, followed by the heavy cream and sweetener. Process for 15-20 seconds.

2. Melt the butter in the microwave and add to the blender along with the coconut oil. Blend until the mixture is smooth and creamy.

3. Using a piping bag, drop fat bombs into a heart mold and place in the freezer for at least 30 minutes. When the fat bombs are set, remove from the mold and enjoy.

4. Keep stored in the freezer.

NUTRITION FACTS (PER SERVING)

Total Carbohydrates: 0g

Dietary Fiber: 0g

Net Cabs: 0g

Protein: 0g

Total Fat: 10g

Calories: 90

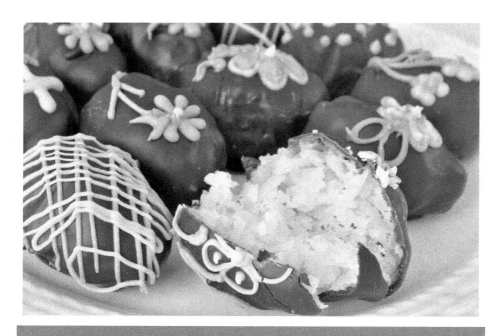

COCONUT EGGS

Preparation time: 25 minutes
Cooking time: 0 minutes
Serves: 12

INGREDIENTS:

- 3 ounces shredded coconut, unsweetened
- 2.5 ounces coconut oil, melted
- 3 tablespoon coconut cream
- 1 tablespoon granulated stevia
- ½ teaspoon vanilla

Chocolate Coating

- 2 ounces coconut oil, melted
- 6 teaspoons cocoa powder
- 2 teaspoons granulated stevia or sugar-free sweetener of choice, to taste

DIRECTIONS:

1. In a small bowl, combine the coconut oil, coconut cream, sweetener, vanilla and shredded coconut.
2. Place the mixture in the fridge for 25-30 minutes. Then shape into egg shape balls and place on a plate lined with wax paper. Return back into the fridge and chill until the eggs have hardened.
3. To prepare the chocolate coating, in a small bowl, whisk the coconut oil, cocoa powder and stevia together until smooth. Coat the eggs thoroughly with chocolate coating and refrigerate until the coating is set.

NUTRITION FACTS (PER SERVING)

Total Carbohydrates: 2g

Dietary Fiber: 1 g

Net Cabs: 1 g

Protein: 1g

Total Fat: 15g

Calories: 143

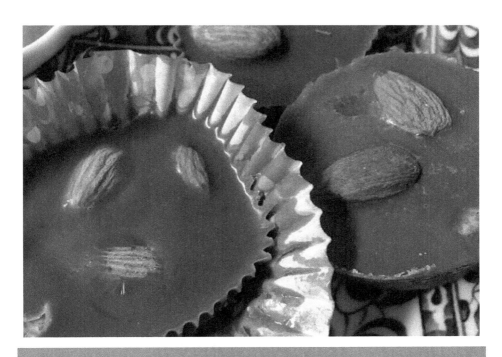

ALMOND FAT BOMBS

Preparation time: 5 minutes

Cooking time: 0 minutes

Serves: 24

INGREDIENTS:

- ½ cup almond butter
- ¼ cup butter
- 2 tablespoons coconut oil
- 1 tablespoon sugar-free maple syrup

DIRECTIONS:

1. Combine the almond butter, coconut oil and butter in a microwave-safe bowl and microwave for 2 minutes until melted, stirring halfway through.
2. Stir in the maple syrup.
3. Spoon the mixture into paper liners designed for candies and freeze for at least 30 minutes until hardened.

NUTRITION FACTS (PER SERVING)

Total Carbohydrates: 2g

Dietary Fiber: 0g

Net Cabs: 1g

Protein: 1g

Total Fat: 6g

Calories: 58

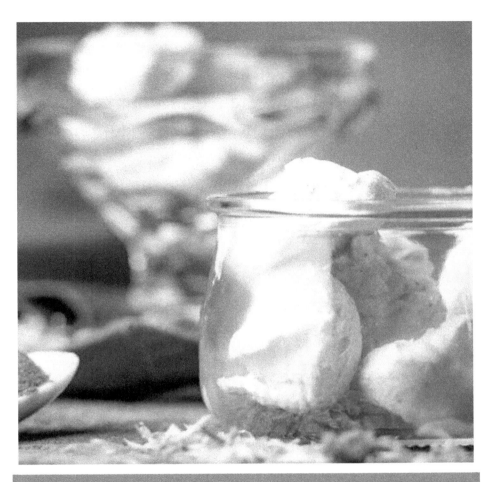

MASCARPONE FAT BOMBS

Preparation time: 5 minutes
Cooking time: 0 minutes
Serves: 10

INGREDIENTS:

- 1/3 cup mascarpone cheese
- 1/3 cup unsweetened coconut flakes
- 1/3 cup coarsely chopped walnuts and/or pecans
- 1 tablespoon Truvia

Coating:

- 4 tablespoons butter
- 2 tablespoons heavy white cream
- 2 tablespoons unsweetened cocoa
- 2 tablespoons Truvia

DIRECTIONS:

1. In a medium bowl, mix the mascarpone, coconut flakes, nuts and sweetener together. Mix well and shape the mixture into small balls. Place on a plate lined with parchment and place in the fridge.

2. Meanwhile, prepare the coating. Combine the butter and heavy cream in a bowl and microwave for 30-35 seconds, stirring once halfway through. Stir in the sweetener and cocoa and mix until well combined.

3. Remove the chilled balls from the fridge and thoroughly coat with the prepared cocoa mixture. Return back to the fridge and let them chill for another 15-20 minutes.

4. Keep stored in the refrigerator.

NUTRITION FACTS (PER SERVING)

Total Carbohydrates: 2g

Dietary Fiber: 0g

Net Cabs: 2g

Protein: 2g

Total Fat: 10g

Calories: 100

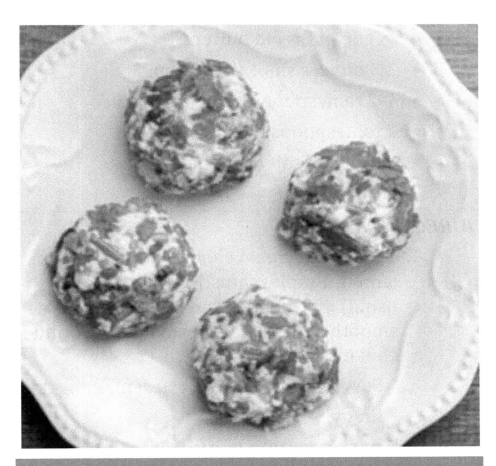

SALMON FAT BOMBS

Preparation time: 5 minutes

Cooking time: 0 minutes

Serves: 15

INGREDIENTS:

- 1 cup cream cheese

- ½ cup grass fed butter
- 3.5 ounces smoked salmon
- 1-2 tablespoons fresh lemon juice
- 2 tablespoons dill, divided
- A pinch of salt (optional)

DIRECTIONS:

1. Place the cream cheese, butter, salmon, lemon, 1 tablespoon dill and salt (if using) in a blender and pulse until smooth and creamy. Form into balls and chill in the fridge.
2. Serve garnished with the remaining dill.
3. Enjoy!

NUTRITION FACTS (PER SERVING)

Total Carbohydrates: 1g

Dietary Fiber: 0g

Net Cabs: 1g

Protein: 3g

Total Fat: 13g

Calories: 117

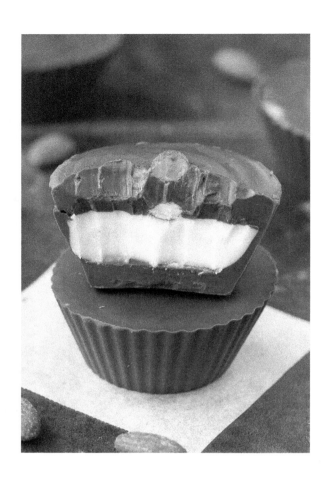

ALMOND CHOCOLATE FAT BOMBS

Preparation time: 10 minutes
Cooking time: 0 minutes
Serves: 16

INGREDIENTS:

- 3/4-1 cup sweetener (or to taste)
- 1/4 cup butter, softened
- 1/4 teaspoon vanilla extract
- 1/4 cup almond milk
- 1 cup almond flour
- 1/2 cup dark chocolate chips
- Chopped pecans (optional)

DIRECTIONS:

1. Combine the almond milk, flour, butter, vanilla extract, chocolate chips and pecans (if using) in a blender or food processor and pulse to reach a smooth consistency.
2. Pour into a mold and chill for 1-2 hours until set.

NUTRITION FACTS (PER SERVING)

Total Carbohydrates: 0g

Dietary Fiber: 0g

Net Cabs: 0g

Protein: 0g

Total Fat: 3g

Calories: 28

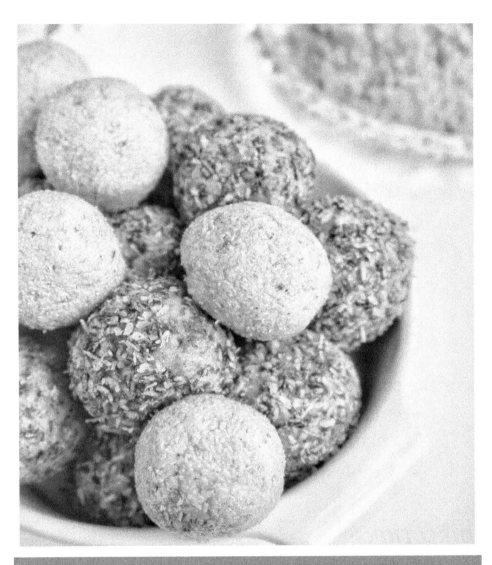

MATCHA TEA FAT BOMBS

Preparation time: 10 minutes

Cooking time: 0 minutes

Serves: 32

INGREDIENTS:

For the truffles:

- 1 cup firm coconut oil (chilled)
- 1 cup creamy coconut butter
- 1/2 cup full fat coconut milk (chilled)
- 1/2 teaspoon matcha green tea powder
- 1/4 teaspoon ground Ceylon cinnamon
- 1/4 teaspoon Himalayan salt
- 1 teaspoon pure vanilla extract
- Sugar substitute (e.g. Stevia) to taste

For the coating:

- 1 cup finely shredded unsweetened coconut
- 1 tablespoon matcha green tea powder

DIRECTIONS:

1. In a large bowl, combine the coconut oil, coconut butter, coconut milk, green tea, Ceylon cinnamon, vanilla, sweetener to taste and salt. Using a hand mixer, mix the ingredients until smooth and creamy.

40

2. Cover and place the bowl in the fridge for an hour.

3. Meanwhile, in a shallow bowl, mix together the shredded coconut and matcha powder. Set aside.

4. Using an ice cream scoop (preferably a small one), shape the chilled mixture into about 30-32 small balls. Roll each ball in the matcha mixture until evenly coated.

5. Place the fat bombs in an airtight container and store in the refrigerator for up to 2 weeks.

6. Enjoy cold or at room temperature.

NUTRITION FACTS (PER SERVING)

Total Carbohydrates: 3g

Dietary Fiber: 2g

Net Cabs: 1g

Protein: 1g

Total Fat: 14g

Calories: 135

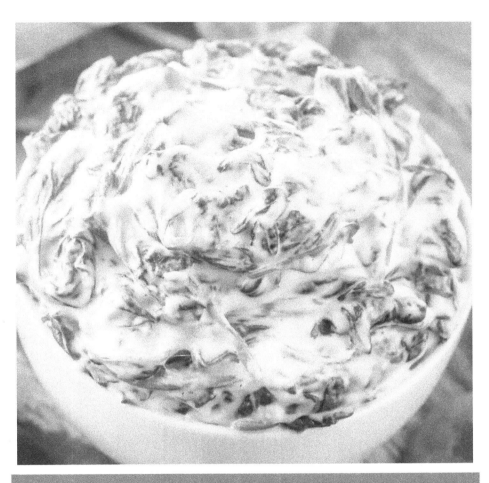

CREAMY SPINACH

Preparation time: 5 minutes
Cooking time: 20 minutes
Serves: 4

INGREDIENTS:

- ½ cup salted butter
- 4 ounces cream cheese
- ½ cup Parmesan cheese, grated
- 15 ounces boxes frozen chopped spinach, thawed

DIRECTIONS:

1. In a microwave safe bowl thaw the spinach, about 12 minutes on the defrost setting. Remove from the microwave and let it stand for 5 minutes. Squeeze with your hands to remove as much liquid as possible.

2. Return the spinach to the bowl. Add the butter and cream cheese and heat in the microwave for 3-4 minutes until butter and cream cheese have melted. Toss well with a tablespoon to coat evenly.

3. Sprinkle the spinach with a handful of grated parmesan cheese and serve.

NUTRITION FACTS (PER SERVING)

Total Carbohydrates: 7g

Dietary Fiber: 3g

Net Cabs: 4g

Protein: 9g

Total Fat: 28g

Calories: 302

Nutty Chocolate Fat Bombs

Preparation time: 5 minutes

Cooking time: 3 minutes

Serves: 2

INGREDIENTS:

- 2 tablespoons hulled sunflower seeds, unsalted
- 2 teaspoons organic toasted coconut flakes, unsweetened
- 1 teaspoons cocoa powder
- 2 tablespoons butter, unsalted
- 2 tablespoons coconut oil
- 1/2 tablespoons honey

DIRECTIONS:

1. Combine the coconut oil and butter in a small saucepan and melt over low heat. Remove from the heat. Let it cool slightly.

2. Mix in the honey, coconut flakes, sunflower seeds and cocoa powder. Pour

the mixture into an ice cube tray and freeze for an hour until hardened.

3. Enjoy.

NUTRITION FACTS (PER SERVING)

Total Carbohydrates: 3g

Dietary Fiber: 1g

Net Cabs: 2g

Protein: 2g

Total Fat: 27g

Calories: 251

Coconut Fennel Fat Bombs

Preparation time: 5 minutes
Cooking time: 0 minutes
Serves: 12

INGREDIENTS:

- ¼ cup coconut oil, softened
- ¼ cup full fat coconut milk
- ¼ cup raw cacao powder
- ¼ cup Swerve sweetener
- 1 teaspoon vanilla extract
- 1 teaspoon ground fennel seeds
- 1/2 teaspoon sea salt
- Coarse sea salt for top

DIRECTIONS:

1. In a medium bowl, mix the coconut oil and coconut milk with a hand mixer until glossy.

2. Mix in the sweetener, cacao, ground fennel, vanilla, and salt. Once the mixture is well combined, transfer to a plastic bag.

3. Gently pipe the creamy mixture into molds and sprinkle a little coarse salt on top. Place the fat bombs in the freezer for at least 1 hour until hardened.

4. Remove them from the molds and store in a plastic bag in the freezer or fridge.

NUTRITION FACTS (PER SERVING)

Total Carbohydrates: 1g

Dietary Fiber: 1g

Net Cabs: 0g

Protein: 1g

Total Fat: 20g

Calories: 172

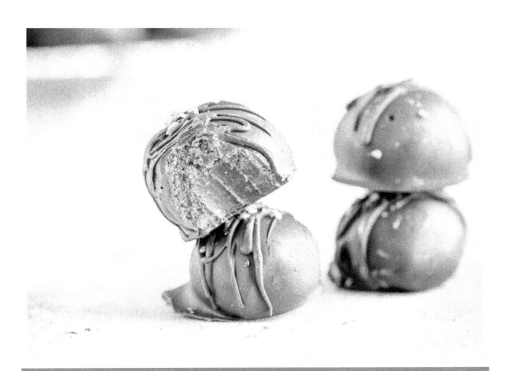

LOW CARB CHOCOLATE TRUFFLES BOMBS

Preparation time: 35 minutes

Cooking time: 0 minutes

Serves: 8

INGREDIENTS:

Ganache Filling

- 5 ounces low carb chocolate

- 2 tablespoons plus 2 teaspoons heavy cream
- ½ teaspoon sugar-free vanilla extract
- 1 ¼ teaspoon chocolate extract

Chocolate Coating

- 2 ounces unsweetened baking chocolate
- ½ ounce cocoa butter
- 1 tablespoon Swerve confectioners sugar
- 1/8 teaspoon stevia extract
- 1/4 teaspoon sugar-free vanilla extract

DIRECTIONS:

1. Melt the chocolate in the microwave. Combine the heavy cream and vanilla in a small microwave safe bowl and heat in the microwave until the mixture is about to boil.

2. Stir in the chocolate extract. Add the melted chocolate, mix well and let it cool for 10 minutes.

3. Cover the bowl with plastic wrap and place in the fridge for at least 3 hours or overnight.

4. Remove from the fridge and bring to room temperature.

5. Shape the ganache mixture into small balls and place on a tray lined with parchment. Transfer to the fridge.

6. Meanwhile start preparing the coating: In the microwave melt the cocoa butter and baking chocolate. Add the vanilla, stevia and confectioners powder and mix well until smooth.

7. Remove the candies from the fridge and roll in the prepared chocolate coating until thoroughly coated.

NUTRITION FACTS (PER SERVING)

Total Carbohydrates: 14g

Dietary Fiber: 7g

Net Cabs: 7g

Protein: 2g

Total Fat: 31g

Calories: 292

Avocado Bacon Fat Bombs

Preparation time: 10 minutes

Cooking time: 15 minutes

Serves: 6

INGREDIENTS:

- ½ large avocado
- ¼ cup butter or ghee, softened at room temperature
- 1 small chili pepper, finely chopped
- ½ small white onion, diced
- 1 tablespoon fresh lime juice
- Freshly ground black or cayenne pepper
- ¼ teaspoon salt
- 4 large slices bacon

DIRECTIONS:

1. Preheat the oven to 375 F⦿.
2. Cut the bacon into strips and place in the baking sheet lined with parchment.

3. Bake in the oven for 15 minutes until golden and crispy. Remove the bacon from the oven and let it cool.

4. Peel the avocado, remove the seed, and cut into quarters. Place in a bowl along with the chili pepper, butter, lime juice and crushed garlic. Add the bacon grease and season with salt and pepper.

5. Using a potato masher, puree the mixture, then and the chopped onions and mix well.

6. Cover the mixture with plastic wrap and refrigerate for 30 minutes.

7. Meanwhile, cut or crush the bacon into small pieces. Shape the chilled mixture into small balls and coat evenly with crumbles and place back into the fridge.

8. Refrigerate for an additional 15 minutes and enjoy.

NUTRITION FACTS (PER SERVING)

Total Carbohydrates: 3g

Dietary Fiber: 1g

Net Cabs: 1g

Protein: 3g

Total Fat: 15g

Calories: 156

Vanilla Fat Bombs

Preparation time: 5 minutes

Cooking time: 10 minutes

Serves: 8

INGREDIENTS:

- 1/4 cup cocoa butter
- 1/4 cup coconut oil
- 9 drops of liquid Stevia
- 1 drop of vanilla extract

DIRECTIONS:

1. Combine the coconut oil and cocoa butter in a small saucepan over low heat.
2. Once melted, remove from the heat. Add the stevia and vanilla extract and stir well. Pour the mixture into a candy mold and freeze for about 1 hour until set.
3. Pop out of the mold and enjoy.
4. Store the candies in an airtight container in the fridge.

NUTRITION FACTS (PER SERVING)

Total Carbohydrates: 0g

Dietary Fiber: 0g

Net Cabs: 0g

Protein: 0g

Total Fat: 14g

Calories: 125

SUMMER

COCONUT LIME FAT BOMBS

Preparation time: 5 minutes

Cooking time: 0 minutes

Makes: 24

INGREDIENTS:

- 1 stick unsalted butter
- 3/4 cup coconut oil
- 1 ounce unsweetened, shredded coconut
- Zest and juice of 2 small limes
- 4 ounces cream cheese, softened
- ¼ cup unsweetened coconut cream
- 1/4 teaspoon vanilla extract
- Sugar-free sweetener of your choice to taste

DIRECTIONS:

1. In a saucepan over medium heat, melt the butter and coconut oil. Once melted,

remove from heat and stir in the lime zest and juice.

2. Stir in the vanilla and shredded coconut. Then add the softened cream cheese and coconut cream. Mix until smooth as possible. If you notice that the cream cheese has separated, don't worry about that as it won't affect the result. Add the sweetener to your taste and mix well.

3. Spoon the mixture into candy molds or candy paper liners and place in the freezer for about an hour. Once they are set, remove from the molds and enjoy.

4. Store the candies in an airtight container in the freezer.

NUTRITION FACTS (PER SERVING)

Total Carbohydrates: 1g

Dietary Fiber: 0g

Net Cabs: 0g

Protein: 1g

Total Fat: 14g

Calories: 122

Cocoa Fat Bombs

Preparation time: 10minutes

Cooking time: 0 minutes

Serves: 20

INGREDIENTS:

- 1 cup mascarpone cheese or full-fat cream cheese
- ¼ cup grass-fed butter or extra virgin coconut oil
- 2 tablespoons MCT oil or more coconut oil
- 2 tablespoons raw cocoa powder, unsweetened
- ¼ cup Erythritol or Swerve, powdered
- 10-15 drops liquid Stevia extract
- ½ teaspoons instant coffee
- 1 teaspoon rum extract

DIRECTIONS:

1. Soften the mascarpone cheese and place in a blender, followed by the MCT oil, butter or coconut oil, cocoa powder and sweeteners.

2. Finally add the instant coffee and pulse to reach a smooth consistency.

3. Pour the mixture into an ice-cube tray about 2 tablespoons for each fat bomb.

4. Freeze for about 3 hours until solid.

NUTRITION FACTS (PER SERVING)

Total Carbohydrates: 1g

Dietary Fiber: 0g

Net Cabs: 1g

Protein: 1g

Total Fat: 8g

Calories: 77

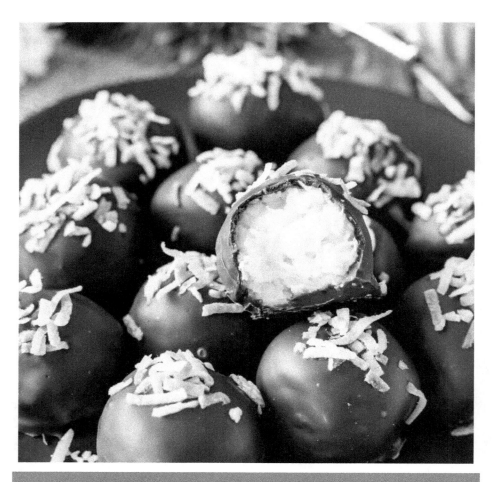

CREAMY COCONUT TRUFFLES

Preparation time: 45 minutes
Cooking time: 0 minutes
Serves: 6

INGREDIENTS:

- ⅓ cup chocolate protein powder
- 2 tablespoons coconut flour
- 2 tablespoons coconut, finely shredded
- 4 tablespoons canned coconut milk
- 1 tablespoon dark cocoa powder
- 1 tablespoon sugar free mini chocolate chips
- ⅔ cup coconut butter, softened (for coating)
- 1 teaspoon coconut oil, softened (for coating)

DIRECTIONS:

1. Place the coconut flour, coconut milk, cocoa powder, shredded coconut, protein powder and chocolate chips in a medium bowl and mix well to combine.

2. Gently spoon the mixture into a medium size mold and transfer to the freezer for 30 minutes.

3. To prepare the coating: In a small bowl, combine the coconut butter and coconut

oil. Melt in the microwave and stir until smooth.

4.   Evenly coat the truffles with the coating mixture and place back into the fridge. Let them refrigerate for another 15-20 minutes.

NUTRITION FACTS (PER SERVING)

Total Carbohydrates: 2g

Dietary Fiber: 1g

Net Cabs: 1g

Protein: 5g

Total Fat: 26g

Calories: 249

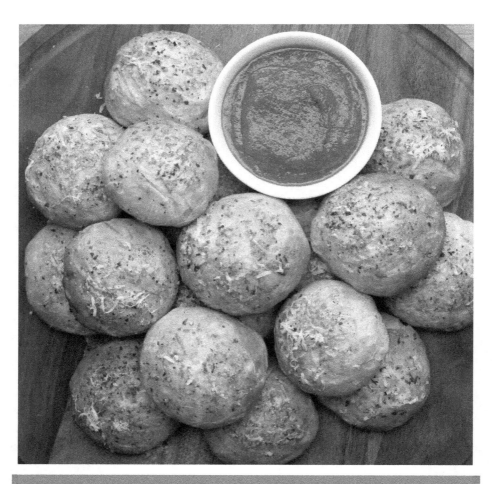

TASTY PIZZA FAT BOMBS

Preparation time: 20 minutes
Cooking time: 0 minutes
Serves: 6

INGREDIENTS:

- 4 ounces cream cheese
- 14 slices Pepperoni
- 8 pitted black olives
- 2 tablespoons sun dried tomato pesto
- 2 tablespoons fresh basil, chopped
- Salt and pepper to taste

DIRECTIONS:

1. In a small bowl, combine the tomato pesto, cream cheese and basil.
2. Thinly slice the olives and pepperoni and add to the bowl. Mix well to combine.
3. Shape the mixture into small balls and place on a serving plate. Chill for 15 minutes and serve garnished with basil leaves and olive.

NUTRITION FACTS (PER SERVING)

Total Carbohydrates: 2g

Dietary Fiber: 0g

Net Cabs: 2g

Protein: 2g

Total Fat: 11g

Calories: 110

LEMON COCONUT FAT BOMBS

Preparation time: 5 minutes

Cooking time: 0 minutes

Serves: 16

INGREDIENTS:

- 7 ounces coconut butter, softened
- ¼ cup extra virgin coconut oil, softened
- Fresh lemon zest from 1-2 lemons
- 15-20 drops Stevia extract or other sweetener to taste
- A pinch of salt

DIRECTIONS:

1. Thoroughly wash the lemons and zest them using a fine grater.

2. In a small bowl, soften the coconut oil and coconut butter. Add the sweetener, pinch of salt and lemon zest. Mix well to combine. Drop about 1 tablespoon of coconut mixture into a silicone candy

mold or candy paper liners and freeze for an hour until they hardened.

3.   Store the done candies in the fridge.

NUTRITION FACTS (PER SERVING)

Total Carbohydrates: 3g

Dietary Fiber: 2

Net Cabs: 1g

Protein: 1g

Total Fat: 12g

Calories: 58

KETO CREAM CHEESE JELLO FAT BOMBS

Preparation time: 10 minutes

Cooking time: 0 minutes

Serves: 8

INGREDIENTS:

- 1 (8 ounce) package of cream cheese
- 1 package of sugar free Jello

DIRECTIONS:

1. Place the unsweetened Jello in a small bowl. Shape the cream cheese into a 16 equal balls.

2. Then roll them in the Jello until evenly coated. Arrange the balls on a plate, cover with plastic wrap and chill in the fridge.

NUTRITION FACTS (PER SERVING)

Total Carbohydrates: 1g

Dietary Fiber: 0 g

Net Cabs: 1g

Protein: 3g

Total Fat: 9g

Calories: 105

GOAT CHEESE TOMATO FAT BOMBS

Preparation time: 10 minutes

Cooking time: 0 minutes

Serves: 7

INGREDIENTS:

- 4 ounce goat cheese
- ½ cup sundried tomatoes
- 1/2 cup pistachios (shelled)
- Salt to taste

DIRECTIONS:

1. Divide the goat cheese into 7 pieces and shape into small balls.
2. Roughly crush the pistachios and sun dried tomatoes and place in a bowl. Season with salt to taste and mix.

3. Coat the cheese balls with the pistachio mixture and refrigerate for at least 15 minutes.

NUTRITION FACTS (PER SERVING)

Total Carbohydrates: 3g

Dietary Fiber: 1g

Net Cabs: 2g

Protein: 7g

Total Fat: 10g

Calories: 125

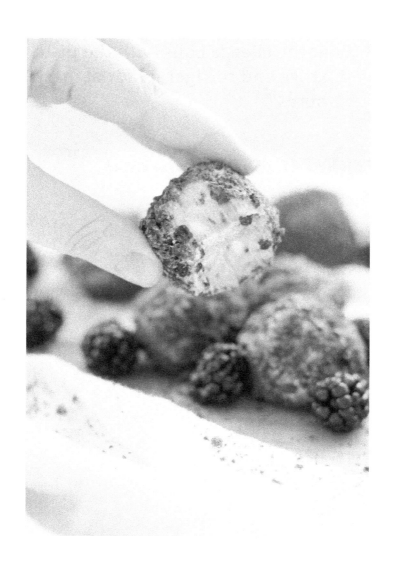

BLACKBERRY CHEESE FAT BOMBS

Preparation time: 10 minutes
Cooking time: 0 minutes
Serves: 10

INGREDIENTS:

- 1/2 cup blackberries (fresh or frozen)
- 2 tablespoons mascarpone cheese
- 1 cup coconut oil
- 1 cup coconut butter
- 1/4 teaspoon vanilla extract
- 1/2 teaspoon lemon juice
- 1/2 teaspoon liquid Stevia
- Stevia to taste

DIRECTIONS:

1. If using frozen blackberries, thaw them in a small bowl.
2. Combine the coconut oil, coconut butter, lemon juice and cheese in a large mixing bowl.
3. Add the blackberries and using a hand mixer, mix them on low until as smooth as possible.
4. Spoon the mixture into a silicone mold and place in the freezer for 30-40 minutes until hardened.

5. Keep the fat bombs stored in the fridge.

NUTRITION FACTS (PER SERVING)

Total Carbohydrates: 3g

Dietary Fiber: 1g

Net Cabs: 2g

Protein: 1g

Total Fat: 41g

Calories: 372

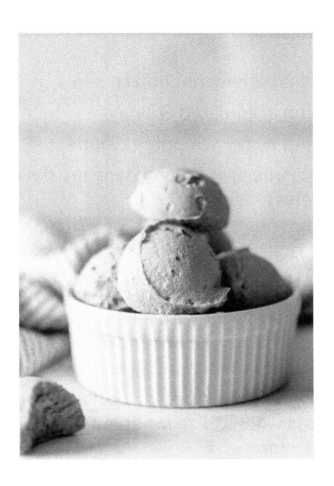

ICE CREAM FAT BOMBS

Preparation time: 10 minutes
Cooking time: 0 minutes
Serves: 10

INGREDIENTS:

- 1 cup cashew nut butter
- 1 cup granulated Stevia
- 1 cup heavy whipping cream
- 3 scoops protein powder (any flavor you prefer)

DIRECTIONS:

1. Place the whipping cream in a mixing bowl and beat with a hand mixer until frothy. With the mixer on low, mix in the protein powder and granulated Stevia.

2. Spoon the mixture into silicone cupcake molds and freeze for about an hour until hardened.

3. When ready to eat, remove from the molds and enjoy.

NUTRITION FACTS (PER SERVING)

Total Carbohydrates: 10g

Dietary Fiber: 2g

Net Cabs: 8g

Protein: 11g

Total Fat: 19g

Calories:250

MANGO CREAM CHEESE FAT BOMBS

Preparation time: 15 minutes

Cooking time: 0 minutes

Serves: 12

INGREDIENTS:

- 1 teaspoon coconut oil
- 2 teaspoon unsalted almond butter
- 1/4 teaspoon cinnamon
- 1 teaspoon unsweetened cocoa powder
- 5 drops stevia
- 1 pinch sea salt

Cheesecake topping

- 1/4 cup mango puree
- 1/2 cup cream cheese
- 1/4 cup unsalted butter
- 1 teaspoon pure vanilla extract
- 1 tablespoon whipping cream

DIRECTIONS:

1. In a small bowl, combine the coconut oil, almond butter, cocoa powder, cinnamon, stevia and sea salt

2. Mix well and spoon into the bottom of the candy molds or ice cube tray.

3. Place in the freezer.

4. In the meantime, place the mango puree, cream cheese, butter, vanilla and heavy cream in a mixing bowl, and whip well using a hand mixer on low, about 5 minutes.

5. Remove the hardened "crusts" from the freezer and top each of them with the prepared topping and return back into the freezer for an hour.

NUTRITION FACTS (PER SERVING)

Total Carbohydrates: 1g

Dietary Fiber: 0g

Net Cabs: 1g

Protein: 1g

Total Fat: 8g

Calories: 77

BLUEBERRY FAT BOMBS

Preparation time: 5 minutes

Cooking time: 3 minutes

Serves: 24

INGREDIENTS:

- 1 cup blueberries
- 1 stick butter
- 3/4 cup coconut oil
- 4 ounces cream cheese, softened
- ¼ cup coconut cream
- Sugar-free sweetener to taste

DIRECTIONS:

1. Place the butter and coconut oil in a small saucepan and melt over low heat. Remove from heat and set aside.

2. Meanwhile, combine the coconut cream, softened cream cheese and berries in a blender and pulse until smooth.

3. Add the melted butter and coconut oil and blend for 15-20 seconds until combined and smooth.

4. Taste and add sugar-free sweetener to your taste. Pour the mixture into molds and freeze for 1-2 hours until they have hardened.

5. Remove from the molds and enjoy.

NUTRITION FACTS (PER SERVING)

Total Carbohydrates: 20g

Dietary Fiber: 18g

Net Cabs: 2g

Protein: 44g

Total Fat: 13g

Calories: 116

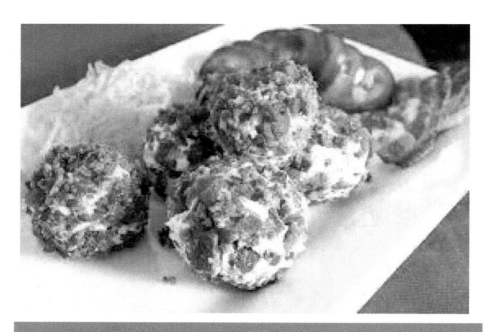

JALAPENO CREAM CHEESE FAT BOMBS

Preparation time: 35 minutes

Cooking time: 0 minutes

Serves: 3

INGREDIENTS:

- 3 ounces cream cheese
- 3 slices bacon
- 1 medium jalapeno pepper
- 1/2 teaspoon dried parsley
- 1/4 teaspoon onion powder

- 1/4 teaspoon garlic powder
- Salt and pepper to taste

DIRECTIONS:

1. Place 3 slices of bacon in a medium skillet and fry until crisp on both sides.
2. Transfer to a plate lined with paper towel and let them cool, reserving the bacon fat.
3. Remove the seeds from the jalapeno pepper and thinly slice it. Place in a small bowl along with the cream cheese and bacon fat. Add the onion powder, garlic powder, parsley, salt and pepper and mix well to combine.
4. Break up the bacon into small pieces and place on a plate.
5. Shape the cream cheese mixture into walnut size balls and coat with the bacon crumbles.
6. Chill the fat bombs for 15-20 minutes and enjoy.

NUTRITION FACTS (PER SERVING)

Total Carbohydrates: 2g

Dietary Fiber: 1g

Net Cabs: 2g

Protein: 5g

Total Fat: 19g

Calories: 207

ALMOND FAT BOMBS

Preparation time: 5 minutes

Cooking time: 0 minutes

Serves: 4

INGREDIENTS:

- ¾ cup melted coconut oil
- ½ cup almond butter
- 60 drops (about 3/8 tsp.) liquid Stevia
- 3 tablespoons cocoa
- 8 tablespoons (1 stick) salted butter, melted

DIRECTIONS:

1. Melt the coconut oil and butter in a saucepan over low heat. Add the almond butter, stevia, cocoa and stir well to combine.

2. Place a silicone mold on a small cookie sheet. Pour about 2 tablespoons of mixture into each of silicone candy molds and place in the freezer for an hour.

3. Once hardened, remove from the molds and serve.

4. Keep the leftovers stored in an airtight container in the freezer.

NUTRITION FACTS (PER SERVING)

Total Carbohydrates: 2g

Dietary Fiber: 0g

Net Cabs: 2g

Protein: 2g

Total Fat: 14 g

Calories: 141

FALL

PEANUT FAT BOMBS

Preparation time: 10 minutes

Cooking time: 0 minutes

Serves: 6

INGREDIENTS:

- 9 ounces of butter
- 2 tablespoons peanut butter
- ¼ cup sugar-free sweetener to taste
- 1/3 cup cocoa
- 1 ounce of heavy cream
- 1 teaspoon vanilla extract

DIRECTIONS:

1. In a microwave safe bowl, melt the butter.
2. Add the peanut butter and mix well.
3. Mix in the cocoa, sweetener, vanilla extract, and heavy cream.

4. Pour the mixture into a candy mold and allow to harden in the freezer for about an hour.

NUTRITION FACTS (PER SERVING)

Total Carbohydrates: 4g

Dietary Fiber: 2g

Net Cabs: 0g

Protein: 2g

Total Fat: 38g

Calories: 350

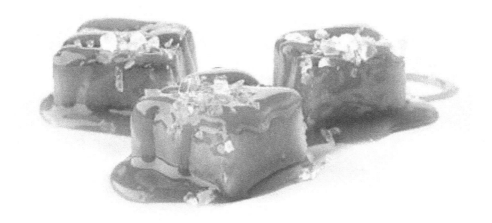

CARAMEL FAT BOMBS

Preparation time: 5 minutes
Cooking time: 0 minutes
Serves: 36

INGREDIENTS:

- 1 cup butter, softened to room temperature
- 1 cup coconut oil
- ¼ cup sour cream
- ¼ cup heavy whipping cream
- Caramel sugar and sweetener to taste

- Coarse ground sea salt

DIRECTIONS:

1. Combine the butter and coconut oil in a mixing bowl and mix well.
2. Add the sour cream, heavy cream, caramel sugar, and sweetener and mix well with a whisk until well combined.
3. Pour the mixture into molds, sprinkle with sea salt and place in the freezer.
4. When the fat bombs become solid, remove from the mold and enjoy.
5. Store them in the fridge.

NUTRITION FACTS (PER SERVING)

Total Carbohydrates: 0g

Dietary Fiber: 0g

Net Cabs: 0g

Protein: 0g

Total Fat: 12g

Calories: 100

Coconut Cinnamon Fat Bombs

Preparation time: 5 minutes

Cooking time: 0 minutes

Serves: 6

INGREDIENTS:

- 4 tablespoons butter, softened
- 4 ounces cream cheese
- 2 tablespoons extra virgin coconut oil
- Dash of cinnamon
- Splash of vanilla extract
- 2 Splenda packets or sugar-free sweetener of your choice, to taste

DIRECTIONS:

1. In a small bowl, combine the butter, cream cheese, and coconut oil.
2. Add the sweetener, cinnamon and vanilla. Mix well until the mixture becomes smooth.

3. Spoon the mixture into a candy mold (any shape) or ice cube tray and place in the freezer for 3-4 hours.

4. Pop the candies out and enjoy.

NUTRITION FACTS (PER SERVING)

Total Carbohydrates: 1 g

Dietary Fiber: 0g

Net Cabs: 0g

Protein: 1g

Total Fat: 18g

Calories: 165

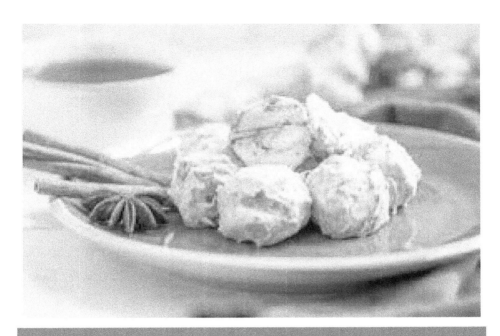

CHAI FAT BOMBS

Preparation time: 5 minutes

Cooking time: 0 minutes

Serves: 15

INGREDIENTS:

- 1 cup coconut oil
- 1 cup heavy cream
- ½ cup butter
- 2 teaspoons cardamom
- 2 teaspoons ginger

- 1 teaspoons cloves
- 1 teaspoons nutmeg
- 10 drops EZ-sweetz (liquid sweetener)
- 1 teaspoon vanilla extract (optional)

DIRECTIONS:

1. Melt the coconut oil, heavy cream and butter in a small saucepan over low heat.
2. Add the sweetener, ginger, cardamom, cloves, nutmeg and vanilla extract and stir well to combine.
3. Pour the mixture into molds and freeze for at least 1 hour. Once they have completely hardened, remove from the molds and enjoy.
4. Keep the candies stored in the fridge.

NUTRITION FACTS (PER SERVING)

Total Carbohydrates: 1g

Dietary Fiber: 0g

Net Cabs: 1g

Protein: 1g

Total Fat: 19g

Calories: 178

CINNAMON BUN FAT BOMBS

Preparation time: 10 minutes

Cooking time: 0 minutes

Serves: 10

INGREDIENTS:

- 1 cup coconut butter
- 1 cup canned coconut milk
- 1 cup unsweetened, shredded coconut
- 1 teaspoon vanilla extract
- ½ teaspoon cinnamon
- ½ teaspoon nutmeg
- 1 teaspoon sugar substitute

DIRECTIONS:

1. Combine all ingredients except for the shredded coconut together in a double boiler or a bowl set over a saucepan of simmering water. Stir until everything is melted and combined.

2. Remove bowl from heat and place in the fridge until the mixture has firmed up and can be rolled into balls.

3. Form the mixture into 1" balls.

4. Roll each ball in the shredded coconut until well coated.

5. Store in the fridge as they will melt at room temperature.

NUTRITION FACTS (PER SERVING)

Total Carbohydrates: 6g

Dietary Fiber: 2g

Net Cabs: 4g

Protein: 1g

Total Fat: 27g

Calories: 259

PUMPKIN PIE FAT BOMBS

Preparation time: 35 minutes

Cooking time: 5 minutes

Serves: 18

INGREDIENTS:

- 3.5 ounces extra dark chocolate
- 2 tablespoons extra virgin coconut oil
- ½ cup coconut butter
- ¼ cup extra virgin coconut oil
- 2 teaspoon pumpkin pie spice mix
- 2 tablespoons powdered Erythritol or Swerve
- ½ cup unsweetened pumpkin puree

DIRECTIONS:

1. Combine the chocolate and coconut oil in a microwave safe bowl and melt in the microwave.

2. Drop about 2 teaspoons of mixture into 16-18 muffin cups and refrigerate for 20 minutes.

3. In a saucepan, combine the coconut oil, coconut butter, pumpkin spice mix, and powdered sweetener. Heat over low heat until melted. Remove from the heat and stir in the pumpkin puree.

4. Remove the muffin cups from the refrigerator and spoon about 2 teaspoons of the pumpkin mixture into each of the cups.

5. Return back to the fridge for at least 1 hour until set.

6. Keep stored in the fridge or freezer as coconut butter and oil get soft at room temperature.

NUTRITION FACTS (PER SERVING)

Total Carbohydrates: 4g

Dietary Fiber: 2g

Net Cabs: 2g

Protein: 1g Total Fat: 11g Calories: 110

ALMOND CINNAMON FAT BOMBS

Preparation time: 5 minutes

Cooking time: 3 minutes

Serves: 4

INGREDIENTS:

- 2 tablespoons coconut oil
- 2 tablespoons almond butter
- 1 tablespoons instant oats
- ¼ teaspoons cinnamon
- 1 tablespoons Stevia

DIRECTIONS:

1. In a small saucepan, melt the coconut oil over low heat. Remove from heat.
2. Add the almond butter to the saucepan followed by the instant oats, cinnamon and stevia. Mix well until smooth.
3. Spoon the mixture into candy molds and place in a freezer for 1-2 hours.
4. Remove from the molds and enjoy.

NUTRITION FACTS (PER SERVING)

Total Carbohydrates: 1g

Dietary Fiber: 0g

Net Cabs: 1g

Protein: 1g

Total Fat: 8g

Calories: 74

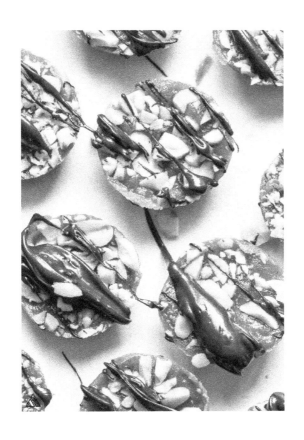

PEANUT BUTTER CHOCOLATE FAT BOMBS

Preparation time: 10 minutes

Cooking time: 30 minutes

Serves: 24

INGREDIENTS:

- 2 tablespoons unsweetened cocoa powder
- 4 tablespoons unsalted butter, softened
- 4 tablespoons peanut butter natural (no sugar added)
- 4 tablespoons coconut oil
- Stevia to taste

DIRECTIONS:

1. In a small bowl, combine the butter, coconut oil, peanut butter, and cocoa powder.
2. Mix until well combined.
3. Spoon the mixture into silicon molds and store in the freezer for 30 minutes.
4. Remove from the molds and enjoy.

NUTRITION FACTS (PER SERVING)

Total Carbohydrates: 1g

Dietary Fiber: 0g

Net Cabs: 1g

Protein: 1g

Total Fat: 6g

Calories: 54

Nutty Fat Bombs

Preparation time: 5 minutes

Cooking time: 5 minutes

Serves: 6

INGREDIENTS:

- 2 ounces cocoa butter
- 2 tablespoons unsweetened cocoa powder
- 2 tablespoons Swerve
- 4 ounces macadamia nuts, chopped
- ¼ cup heavy cream or coconut oil (for dairy free option)

DIRECTIONS:

1. Fill a saucepan halfway with water and bring to a boil over high heat. Place the cocoa butter in a bowl and set it over the boiling water. Once melted, stir in the cocoa powder.

2. Add the sweetener and macadamia nuts. Mix well and remove from the heat.

3. Whisk in the heavy cream or coconut oil.

4. Let the mixture cool and then pour into silicone molds or paper liners designed for candies.

5. Place in the refrigerator for about an hour until hardened.

NUTRITION FACTS (PER SERVING)

Total Carbohydrates: 3g

Dietary Fiber: 0g

Net Cabs: 3g

Protein: 3g

Total Fat: 28g

Calories: 367

VANILLA COCONUT FAT BOMBS

Preparation time: 5 minutes

Cooking time: 0 minutes

Serves: 5

INGREDIENTS:

- 1/2 cup of vanilla protein powder
- 1/4 cup of flaked coconut
- 1/4 cup of coconut flour
- 1/4 cup of coconut milk
- 1 tablespoons butter
- 1 ounce dark chocolate (85% cacao) or sesame seeds

DIRECTIONS:

1. In a medium bowl, combine the coconut milk, coconut flour, softened butter, vanilla and flaked coconut.
2. Mix well and shape the mixture into small balls.

3. Melt the chocolate in the microwave. Coat the balls with melted chocolate and refrigerate before serving.
4. Alternatively you can coat the balls with sesame seeds.

NUTRITION FACTS (PER SERVING)

Total Carbohydrates: 3g

Dietary Fiber: 2g

Net Cabs: 1g

Protein: 9g

Total Fat: 9g

Calories: 123

APPLE CINNAMON FAT BOMBS

Preparation time: 5 minutes

Cooking time: 5 minutes

Serves: 12

INGREDIENTS:

- 2 medium organic green apples, cored and thinly sliced
- 2 tablespoons coconut oil
- 1 teaspoon cinnamon
- 1 (5.4 ounce) can coconut cream
- 1/2 cup coconut butter
- 20 drops of Stevia
- Pinch sea salt

DIRECTIONS:

1. Melt the coconut oil in a skillet over medium heat.

2. Add the apples and cook until they become tender. Sprinkle with cinnamon and stir well to coat.

3. Add the coconut cream, coconut butter, sautéed apples, stevia, and sea salt to a blender and pulse to reach a smooth consistency.

4. Pour the mixture into silicone molds (any size and shape) and freeze until hardened. Remove from the molds and enjoy.

5. Store the leftovers in the refrigerator.

NUTRITION FACTS (PER SERVING)

Total Carbohydrates: 14g

Dietary Fiber: 2g

Net Cabs: 12g

Protein: 0g

Total Fat: 12g

Calories: 168

CHOCOLATE AND WALNUT FAT BOMBS

Preparation time: 5 minutes

Cooking time: 0 minutes

Serves: 14

INGREDIENTS:

- 5 ounces coconut oil
- 1 ounce cocoa powder
- 1 tablespoon granulated stevia, or sweetener of choice to taste
- 1 ounce walnut pieces
- 1 tablespoon tahini paste

DIRECTIONS:

1. Melt the coconut oil in a saucepan over low heat.
2. Add the chopped walnuts, cocoa powder, stevia and tahini paste. Mix well to combine. Let the mixture cool.
3. Pour into a silicone mold or ice cube tray and place in the refrigerator until the

candies have almost hardened. Top each of the candies with a half piece of walnut and place back in the fridge until completely hardened.

NUTRITION FACTS (PER SERVING)

Total Carbohydrates: 1g

Dietary Fiber: 1g

Net Cabs: 0g

Protein: 1g

Total Fat: 12g

Calories: 111

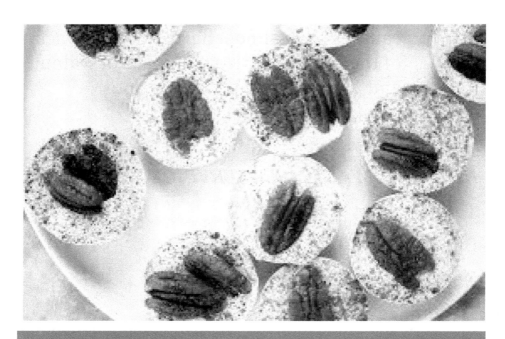

SPICY PUMPKIN FAT BOMBS

Preparation time: 10 minutes

Cooking time: 6 minutes

Serves: 10

INGREDIENTS:

- 4 tablespoons unsalted butter, softened
- 2 tablespoons coconut oil
- ½ cup pumpkin
- ¼ teaspoon ginger
- 1/8 teaspoon clove

- ¼ teaspoon nutmeg
- ¼ teaspoon cinnamon
- Liquid Stevia to taste

DIRECTIONS:

1. Melt the coconut oil in the microwave and add to the butter. Mix well until light and creamy.
2. Add the pumpkin and mix well until smooth. Whisk in the stevia and spices. Using a spoon, drop the mixture on the wax paper and chill for 15 minutes.
3. Then remove from the fridge, form the chilled pieces into balls and place back in the fridge for 1-2 hours.

NUTRITION FACTS (PER SERVING)

Total Carbohydrates: 1g

Dietary Fiber: 0g

Net Cabs: 1g

Protein: 2g

Total Fat: 10g

Calories: 99

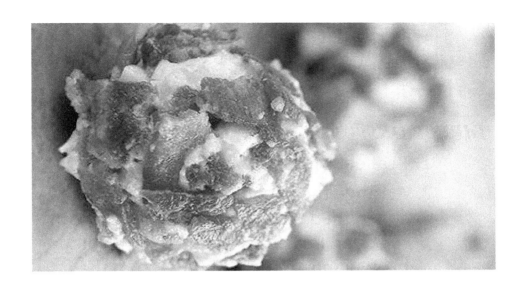

WINTER

EGG AND BACON FAT BOMBS

Preparation time: 10 minutes

Cooking time: 15 minutes

Serves: 6

INGREDIENTS:

- 2 large organic eggs
- 1/3 cup butter, softened
- 2 teaspoons mayonnaise
- Freshly ground black pepper

- ¼ tsp salt or more to taste
- 4 large slices bacon

DIRECTIONS:

1. Preheat the oven to 375▯ F.

2. Arrange the bacon slices on a baking sheet lined with parchment and bake in the oven for 12-15 minutes until golden brown and crispy. Remove from the oven and let them cool. Reserve the bacon grease.

3. Put the eggs in a small pot of water, add a pinch of salt and bring to a boil over medium-high heat. Then reduce the heat to medium and cook for about 10 minutes until the eggs are hard-boiled.

4. Transfer the eggs to a bowl of cold water. When they become cool enough to handle, peel the eggs out of the shells. Cut into quarters and place in a small bowl. Add the butter and mayonnaise and mash with a fork. Mix in the bacon grease and season with the salt and pepper.

5. Chill the mixture for about 30 minutes. Meanwhile crumble the baked bacon into small pieces.

6. When ready to shape fat balls, remove the mixture from the fridge. Using a spoon, shape the mixture into 6 balls and coat with bacon crumbles.

7. Serve immediately. Store the leftover in an airtight container the fridge.

NUTRITION FACTS (PER SERVING)

Total Carbohydrates: 0g

Dietary Fiber: 0g

Net Cabs: 0g

Protein: 5g

Total Fat: 18g

Calories: 185

Coconut Fudge Fat Bombs

Preparation time: 20 minutes

Cooking time: 0 minutes

Serves: 6

INGREDIENTS:

- 1 cup coconut oil, softened
- ¼ cup full fat coconut milk
- ¼ cup organic cocoa powder
- 1 drop of liquid stevia
- 1 teaspoon vanilla extract
- ½ teaspoon almond extract
- ½ teaspoon Celtic sea salt

DIRECTIONS:

1. Combine the coconut milk and coconut oil in a medium bowl and beat with a mixer on medium or high for 5-7 minutes until smooth and glossy.
2. Add the sweetener, vanilla, almond extract, salt and cocoa powder and mix

on medium until well blended. Taste and add another drop of stevia, if desire.

3. Place a sheet of parchment or wax paper along the inside of a loaf pan. Pour the mixture into the prepared pan and chill in the freezer for about 30 minutes until set.

4. Taking the edges of the parchment, remove the fudge from the pan and transfer to a cutting board. Cut the fudge into small squares using a sharp knife.

5. Place the pieces in an airtight container and store in the freezer.

NUTRITION FACTS (PER SERVING)

Total Carbohydrates: 1g

Dietary Fiber: 1g

Net Cabs: 1g

Protein: 0gg

Total Fat: 20g

Calories: 172

CINNAMON AND COCONUT FAT BOMBS

Preparation time: 10 minutes

Cooking time: 5 minutes

Serves: 12

INGREDIENTS:

- 1 cup almond butter
- 1 cup full fat coconut milk
- 1 teaspoon vanilla extract
- 1/2 teaspoon nutmeg
- 1/2 teaspoon cinnamon
- 1 teaspoon Stevia powder extract (or to taste)
- 1 cup unsweetened, shredded coconut

DIRECTIONS:

1. Fill a medium saucepan halfway with cold water and bring to a boil over medium-high heat. Combine the almond butter, coconut milk, cinnamon, nutmeg,

vanilla and Stevia in a glass bowl and set over the saucepan.

2. Stir the mixture, until the almond butter is melted. Remove the bowl from the heat.

3. Let the mixture cool and refrigerate for 20-25 minutes, until the mixture becomes hard enough to shape into balls.

4. Using your hands, shape into small balls and toss in the shredded coconut, until evenly coated.

5. Arrange the balls on a serving plate and chill in the fridge for about an hour before serving.

NUTRITION FACTS (PER SERVING)

Total Carbohydrates: 13g

Dietary Fiber: 8g

Net Cabs: 5g

Protein: 3g

Total Fat: 34g

Calories: 341

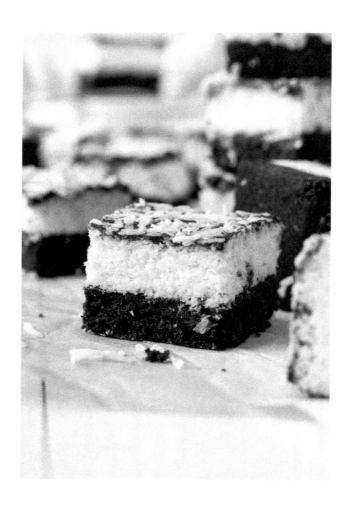

COCONUT BROWNIE

Preparation time: 15 minutes
Cooking time: 25 minutes
Serves: 10

INGREDIENTS:

- ¾ cup coconut butter, melted
- ⅓ cup full fat coconut cream
- 2 tablespoons grass-fed butter, melted
- 1 pastured egg
- 2 teaspoons vanilla extract
- 5 tablespoons cacao powder
- 3/4 cup granulated Stevia
- ¼ teaspoons sea salt
- ¼ teaspoon baking soda

DIRECTIONS:

1. Preheat oven to 350 F▢. Place the cacao powder, baking soda, Stevia, and salt in a small bowl and set aside.

2. Combine the coconut butter, coconut cream and grass-fed butter in a mixing bowl and beat until smooth and creamy.

3. Beat in the egg and vanilla extract. Then mix in the cacao mixture. Beat until there are no lumps in the batter.

4. Coat a 6x6 baking pan with oil. Pour the batter into the pan and bake in the oven

for 22-25 minutes until the edges of the brownie become dark brown.

5. Remove from the oven and let it cool. Then refrigerate the brownie for about 30 minutes before cutting and serving.

NUTRITION FACTS (PER SERVING)

Total Carbohydrates: 1g

Dietary Fiber: 0g

Net Cabs: 1g

Protein: 1g

Total Fat: 20g

Calories: 184

Peppermint Fat Bombs

Preparation time: 10 minutes

Cooking time: 0 minutes

Serves: 6

INGREDIENTS:

- 4.5 ounces coconut oil melted
- 1 tablespoons granulated stevia, or sweetener of choice, to taste
- ¼ teaspoons peppermint extract
- 2 tablespoons cocoa powder

DIRECTIONS:

1. In a small saucepan melt the coconut oil. Mix in the peppermint extract and stevia.
2. Spoon half of the coconut oil into silicone molds and chill in the refrigerator. This will be the white layer of the fat bombs.
3. Once they have hardened, remove from the fridge. Add 2 tablespoons of cocoa powder to the remaining half of mixture

and mix until smooth. Pour over the hardened white parts of candies.

4. Return back to the refrigerator and chill for at least an hour.

NUTRITION FACTS (PER SERVING)

Total Carbohydrates: 1g

Dietary Fiber: 1g

Net Cabs: 1g

Protein: 1gg

Total Fat: 21g

Calories: 188

MINT CHOCOLATE FUDGE

Preparation time: 45 minutes

Cooking time: 0 minutes

Serves: 24

INGREDIENTS:

- 1 ½ cups coconut oil
- 1 ¼ cups nut or seed butter
- ½ cup sweetener (liquid or granulated)
- ½ cup dried parsley flakes
- 2 teaspoons vanilla
- 1 teaspoons peppermint extract
- ¼ teaspoons salt
- 1 cup melted dark (75%) chocolate

DIRECTIONS:

1. Place the coconut oil in a small saucepan and heat over medium heat until melted.

2.	Pour into a blender along with the butter, sweetener, parsley flakes, vanilla, peppermint extract and melted chocolate. Pulse for 30-45 seconds until smooth.

3.	Pour the mixture into a shamrock mold and place in the freezer for at least 1 hour until hardened.

4.	Remove from the freezer and enjoy.

5.	Store the fudge in the refrigerator.

NUTRITION FACTS (PER SERVING)

Total Carbohydrates: 7g

Dietary Fiber: 1g

Net Cabs: 6g

Protein: 3g

Total Fat: 25g

Calories: 251

Orange chocolate Cheesecake Fat Bombs

Preparation time: 5 minutes

Cooking time: 0 minutes

Serves: 12

INGREDIENTS:

For the Chocolate

- 12

DIRECTIONS:

1. In a small saucepan, melt the butter and coconut oil.
2. Remove from the heat. Add the sea salt and cocoa powder and mix well.
3. Stir in the orange extract and sweetener to your taste.
4. To prepare the cheesecake filling: In a mixing bowl, combine the cream cheese, butter, orange juice and zest, and salt and

mix with a hand mixer until smooth and creamy.

5. Fill the silicone molds with a thin layer of chocolate mixture and freeze for 15-20 minutes until set.

6. Remove from the freezer and top with cheesecake mixture. Spoon the remaining chocolate mixture on the top and return the molds back to the freezer. Let them freeze for 1-2 hours and enjoy.

7. Store in a resealable plastic bag in the fridge.

NUTRITION FACTS (PER SERVING)

Total Carbohydrates: 3g

Dietary Fiber: 1g

Net Cabs: 2g

Protein: 1g

Total Fat: 19g

Calories: 177

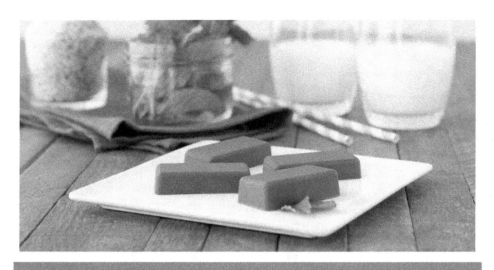

HEMP AND PEPPERMINT FAT BOMBS

Preparation time: 35 minutes

Cooking time: 0 minutes

Serves: 16

INGREDIENTS:

- ¾ cup coconut butter, melted
- 3 tablespoons coconut oil, melted
- 3 tablespoons hemp seeds
- ¼ teaspoon peppermint extract
- 2 tablespoons organic cocoa powder
- 5-8 drops of liquid stevia

DIRECTIONS:

1. Melt the coconut butter and 1 tablespoon of coconut oil in the microwave.

2. Mix in the peppermint extract and hemp seeds. Spoon the mixture into the molds, filling about 3/4 full. Freeze for about 30 minutes until set.

3. In a small bowl, combine 2 tablespoon of melted coconut oil, liquid stevia and cocoa powder.

4. Remove the candies from the freezer and drizzle with the prepared cocoa mixture.

5. Return back to the freezer and allow to harden for about an hour.

6. Pop out of the molds and enjoy.

7. Keep stored in a resalable plastic bag in the fridge.

NUTRITION FACTS (PER SERVING)

Total Carbohydrates: 4g

Dietary Fiber: 3g

Net Cabs: 1g

Protein: 2g

Total Fat: 11g

Calories: 121

Cinnamon Ginger Fat Bombs

Preparation time: 5 minutes

Cooking time: 0 minutes

Serves: 12

INGREDIENTS:

- 4 ounces toasted desiccated coconut
- 2 ounces coconut oil
- 2 ounces butter
- 1 teaspoon cinnamon
- 1 vanilla bean scraped
- 1 tablespoons freshly grated ginger
- 1 teaspoon stevia (or other sweetener)
- Pinch of sea salt

DIRECTIONS:

1. Melt the butter and coconut oil over low heat.
2. Add the coconut, cinnamon, ginger, vanilla, stevia and sea salt. Mix well to

151

combine. Pour the mixture into silicone candy molds and place in the freezer for an hour, until hardened.

3. Remove from the molds and enjoy.
4. Store the leftovers in the fridge.

NUTRITION FACTS (PER SERVING)

Total Carbohydrates: 1g

Dietary Fiber: 0g

Net Cabs: 1g

Protein: 0g

Total Fat: 9g

Calories: 79

KETO CUSTARD RECIPE

Preparation time: 5 minutes

Cooking time: 0 minutes

Serves: 24

INGREDIENTS:

- 4 cups of coconut milk (canned)
- 1 pound unsalted butter or ghee
- 1 cup coconut oil or lard
- 3 tablespoons of plain gelatin
- 11 teaspoons xylitol or 14 teaspoons erythritol
- 10 egg yolks
- 2-3 teaspoons vanilla extract
- 1 cup unsweetened, shredded coconut (optional)

DIRECTIONS:

1. In a large saucepan over low heat, combine the coconut milk, coconut oil,

unsalted butter, gelatin and sweetener. Mix well until the gelatin has dissolved, about 1-2 minutes.

2. Separate the egg yolks and whisk in a large bowl until light and frothy. When the coconut mixture is heated through and it is about to boil, slowly stir in the beaten yolks a little at a time.

3. Stir the mixture constantly until it begins to thicken, about 1-2 minutes.

4. Remove the pan from the heat and place in cold water. Let it cool slightly. At this point, add the vanilla and stir well.

5. Ladle the mixture into dessert bowls, sprinkle with shredded coconut and place in the refrigerator for 1-2 hours.

NUTRITION FACTS (PER SERVING)

Total Carbohydrates: 5g

Dietary Fiber: 1g

Net Cabs: 4g

Protein: 2g

Total Fat: 37g

Calories: 349

PECAN AND WHITE CHOCOLATE FAT BOMBS

Preparation time: 5 minutes

Cooking time: 0 minutes

Serves: 26

INGREDIENTS:

- 1/3 cup coconut oil
- 1/3 cup coconut butter
- 1/3 cup finely chopped cocoa butter (about 1.5 ounces)
- 2 tablespoon powdered erythritol or other powdered sugar substitute, optional
- Liquid sugar substitute to equal 1/4 cup sugar, to taste
- 1 teaspoon sugar-free vanilla extract
- Pinch of salt
- 1 cup lightly toasted pecan halves
-

DIRECTIONS:

1. Line a square baking pan with parchment and place in the fridge to chill.

2. In a glass bowl, combine the coconut oil, coconut butter, and cocoa butter. Set over a medium saucepan filled halfway with simmering water. Alternatively, you may use a double broiler.

3. Stir in the vanilla, sweeteners and pecans. Season the mixture with salt and mix until well combined.

4. Pour the mixture onto the chilled baking pan and transfer to the freezer. Let it freeze for at least 1 hour.

5. Once hardened, remove from the freezer and cut into pieces. Store the candies in an airtight container in the fridge.

6.

NUTRITION FACTS (PER SERVING)

Total Carbohydrates: 1g

Dietary Fiber: 0g

Net Cabs: 1g

Protein: 0g

Total Fat: 10g

Calories: 92

CINNAMON ICE CREAM FAT BOMBS

Preparation time: 10 minutes

Cooking time: 6 minutes

Serves: 10

INGREDIENTS:

- 4 egg yolks
- 2 ½ cups heavy whipping cream, divided
- 2/3 cup crème fraiche or sour cream
- ½ teaspoon Stevia extract
- 2 teaspoon cinnamon
- ¼ teaspoon nutmeg

DIRECTIONS:

1. Separate the egg yolks and place in a double boiler along with 1 ½ cups of the heavy cream. Place the boiler over medium heat for a couple of minutes. Add the nutmeg, cinnamon, and sweetener to the custard and remove from the heat. Let it cool and chill in the fridge.

159

2. To the chilled mixture, add the crème fraiche or sour cream and the remaining 1 cup of heavy cream. Mix with a hand mixer until smooth and creamy.

3. Drop into Christmas tree molds and freeze for at least 1 hour.

4. Once it is completely set, remove from the molds and enjoy.

NUTRITION FACTS (PER SERVING)

Total Carbohydrates: 1g

Dietary Fiber: 0g

Net Cabs: 1g

Protein: 2g

Total Fat: 40g

Calories: 363

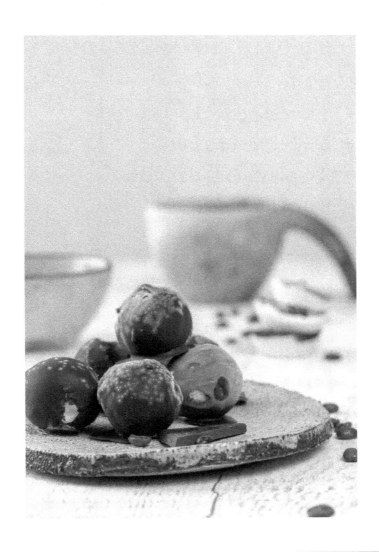

COFFEE AND CHOCOLATE FAT BOMBS

Preparation time: 3 minutes
Cooking time: 5 minutes
Serves: 4

INGREDIENTS:

- 4 tablespoons coconut oil
- 6 tablespoons butter
- 2 tablespoons dark cocoa powder
- 8 ounces coffee

DIRECTIONS:

1. Melt the butter and coconut oil in a small saucepan over low heat.
2. Add the cocoa power and stir well until there are no lumps.
3. Spoon about 4 tablespoon of mixture into each of the silicone cupcake molds and place in the freezer for about 30 minutes.
4. Remove from the molds. Place 1 fat bomb in the bottom of the coffee cup and pour the coffee over.
5. You may add sweetener or heavy cream on top. Stir to combine and enjoy.

NUTRITION FACTS (PER SERVING)

Total Carbohydrates: 2g

Dietary Fiber: 1g

Net Cabs: 1g

Protein: 0g

Total Fat: 31g

Calories: 275

CPSIA information can be obtained
at www.ICGtesting.com
Printed in the USA
BVHW040607080321
601991BV00008B/424

9 781801 562577